# Healing a B[roken Heart]

*The Grand Canyon was not punished b[y the winds].*
*In fact, it was created by them. We a[lso have the]*
*power to weather life's toughest storn[s. Without the]*
*Grand Canyon from the windstorm, we would never have seen the beauty of*
*its carvings.*

Elisabeth Kubler-Ross and David Kessler

Our bodies have an infinite wisdom in healing our physical bodies. When we cut our finger, we don't have to tell our body what to do to heal the cut. It is capable of mending itself.

Healing the grief of a broken heart is another matter. Grief is more than sadness. Grief is a loss. Something of value is gone. Grief is an intense loss that breaks our heart.

Over time, unhealed grief becomes anger, resentment, blame, righteousness, and/or remorse. We become someone we are not. Healing the heart is necessary if we want to move forward with our lives in peace and joy.

It takes courage to move through the grief and all the emotions buried deep within. There are reasons why we sometimes hold onto the pain.

* Sometimes we hold onto the pain to remain "connected" to that which caused our pain ... the death of a loved one, the ending of something we did not want to end.

* Sometimes we hold onto the pain because we cannot or will not forgive. When we are not able to forgive those that hurt us, we remain connected to them.

* Sometimes we hold onto the pain because we do not know how to ... how to let go, how to move on, how to heal the pain of the heart.

* Sometimes we hold onto the pain because we are afraid if we let the pain go, we are letting the loved one go as well. If we let go, we will forget and we do not want to forget. If we let go, maybe they won't come back.

* Sometimes our pain is our identity. Who would we be without our pain?

* Sometimes it is easier to stay in the pain than do anything about it.

* Sometimes we hold onto the pain because we feel if we heal our pain it is letting someone else "off the hook" for creating our pain.

* Sometimes we hold onto the pain because we benefit from a pay-off to remain in the pain; pay-offs of blaming, avoiding, feeling sorry for ourselves, and/or staying angry.

When we hurt ourselves physically, healing can take place with or without any effort on our part. (This is assuming the body and the environment are healthy.) Unfortunately, a broken heart and emotional pain are not the same. Healing the heart, healing emotional hurts do require effort on our part. Time does not heal all.

To heal a broken heart, the dysfunctional beliefs must be identified, acknowledged, addressed, resolved, removed, and healed. The most effective method I have found to do so is EFT Tapping.

# Dear Diary

Friday, October 2, 2015

Dear Diary,

I should tell Roger, "Three strikes, you're out!"

Roger and Stephanie are determined that I meet an incredible guy and live happily ever after. Well, to date, I haven't met an incredible guy nor have I ever had the fulfilling and satisfying relationship that Roger and Stephanie have.

Tonight, they, and when I say "they," I mean Roger, have invited yet another man for me to meet at their home. The first three men were such duds, I am not looking forward to meeting the 4th of Roger's single college buddies.

When Stephanie invited me to dinner, I declined the invitation. Stephanie can be persuasive at times. Today was one of those times. She promised me that Matt is different than the other men that Roger has introduced to me. She thinks I will like him. Reluctantly, I gave in.

Saturday, October 3, 2015

Dear Diary,

I was pleasantly surprised last night. I had a great time and did enjoy Matt. He is different than any of the other men that Roger has introduced me to. He is tall, dark, and handsome and, actually, quite sweet. He has an easiness about him that made me feel comfortable around him even though we just met.

He works for a motivational speaker as part of the advance team handling marketing, sales, and logistics for events around the United States. The speaker doesn't do any events at the end of the year, so Matt is now back at the headquarters. He isn't sure if they will send him out on the road again or keep him at the headquarters next year.

And, yes, we are getting together again. He asked if I would like to go hiking and to breakfast tomorrow. He's picking me up at 4:30 a.m. Fortunately, I am an early riser.

I think what impressed me last night about Matt was his kindness and graciousness. He seemed well-educated, spoke elegantly, and had a genuineness about him that is intriguing.

Why isn't this dude in a relationship or married? Is he too good to be true? That makes me a little leery. I've been burned before by men who have been too good to be true. It is definitely a question on my checklist of questions to find out tomorrow.

Sunday, October 4, 2015

Dear Diary,

I had a great time with Matt today hiking. It's fun to be with an athletic guy who participates in sports instead of just watching them on TV. He did have plans after breakfast to watch the football games at Roger's house with some of their other college buddies.

He texted me this afternoon that he had a wonderful time this morning and would like to get together Wednesday night if I was available. I thought of not being available, playing hard to get, then decided I would rather spend time with him than to play games. I texted back that I was available. He responded back, "Great. Dress causal. I'll pick you up at 6 p.m."

I did ask him about previous relationships and marriage. He did marry his college sweetheart after they both graduated from college. She ended up having an affair and decided she would rather be with the other man. Matt says the other guy was better-looking (which I don't know how that could be possible) and had a trust fund. Apparently the divorce was amiable. She didn't want anything other than what was obviously hers like her clothes, car, and savings account before they married.

He seems healed from the divorce and not scarred. If my husband had an affair with a wealthy woman and left me for her, I don't know if I could be so passive about it. Is "passive" the right word? I don't know him well enough to know if he's truly healed or if it is just repressed.

I found photos of his wife and the whole story of their courtship, engagement, and marriage on his Facebook page. I'm surprised he still has everything on his Facebook page. I think it if was me, I would have deleted anything about the ex.

He was cute in college. There are photos of Roger and Matt playing basketball. Matt towered over Roger! He had a scholarship to play basketball in college, otherwise he would not have been able to afford to attend college. He must have been a good player to have secured a scholarship out of high school that paid for all four years of his college education.

Interesting guy. I like him. I laugh a lot when I am with him. We seem to have a lot in common. We are both athletic and on our days off prefer to spend it riding a bike or hiking a mountain or doing anything that keeps us active.

We are both single without children nor do either of us have an overwhelming urge to be a parent. We are both first-born and have siblings, one brother and one sister. He majored in Business Marketing. I majored in Business Administration. We both have been at our jobs since college and enjoy the companies we work for.

I'm looking for a flaw here. There don't seem to be any. I'm looking for the wrinkle that could trip me up. There don't seem to be any at this point.

At lunch today Stephanie wanted an update. I told her there really wasn't anything to talk about other than we hiked this morning and had breakfast. She didn't believe me. I probably wouldn't believe me either. I don't want to talk about it yet.

Thursday, October 8, 2015

Dear Diary,

Is this guy for real? Matt texted me yesterday to meet him on the boardwalk at the beach. We walked a little on the boardwalk then he took my hand, pulled me onto the sand, and we jogged down toward the water. I noticed a fire in one of the fire rings and a picnic basket.

Well, blow me over! Matt had built the fire and it was our picnic basket! I have never had anyone do anything like this for me. How special I felt. We had a wonderful evening chatting into the late hours of the night.

I think I'm falling for this man. He is incredibly attentive, a great conversationalist, and a sexy kisser. To reciprocate, I asked him out for Saturday. He said he had to go out of town for a few days for work and asked if we could meet in a week, next Wednesday, the 14th.

That worked for me. I have no clue what we're going to do though. I told him I would text him instructions on Tuesday. Help! What am I going to do? It has to be something special since the picnic last night was incredible. I will look online to see if I can find anything fun and special to do Wednesday night.

Saturday, October 10, 2015

Dear Diary,

Along with a hundred other people, Stephanie and I attended a yoga meet-up group this morning basking in the early morning sunlight at the beach. On the next blanket over was an unusual man. Very limber. Very fit. After class he struck up a conversation with me. Unfortunately, Stephanie was on a timetable and we had to leave. He said he would see me next Saturday if we come back to class. Way cool!

Sunday, October 11, 2015

Dear Diary,

I have a great event for Matt and I to attend Wednesday night. It's called Taste of Coronado. The notice said, "Spend a night with us on Coronado Island, indulging your senses and enjoying amazing bites prepared by our local chefs. Take a culinary trip around the world, sampling from our local bistros. This will be a night to remember so come and bring your friends." I think I will go… and bring a friend!

This could be fun. He surprised me with a meal. I will top that with food from around the world! I bought tickets for the two of us.

Tuesday, October 13, 2015

Dear Diary,

Bright and early this morning, I received a text from Matt asking how he should dress for tonight. I like that he remembered our date. I like that he already texted me before I was even out of bed! This guy is an early riser.

I responded and told him casual. I also gave him the address and time where we would meet. I included a P.S.: Bring your bike.

Sunday, November 29, 2015

Dear Diary,

Wow, it's been more than 6 weeks since I last wrote. The relationship between Matt and I has heated up. We talk every day and see each other at least twice a week, if not more. We just spent the Thanksgiving weekend together. Four days flew by. We headed to Lake Tahoe to enjoy the season, cold weather, and to hike.

It is so easy to be with Matt. We fit together like a baseball in a baseball mitt. I think I have found my Mr. Right. I can see myself as his wife. I could spend the rest of my life with Matt and be happy and content. I feel a contentment with Matt that I have never felt with anyone else. I feel as if I have been blessed and that I am the luckiest woman in the world.

I have never felt cherished before. Matt makes me feel cherished, valued, and loved.

When I had lunch with Stephanie today, I told her that I finally understood what she and Roger have together because I thought Matt and I had that same feeling.

Tall, dark, and handsome is only half the package. Aware, present, and understanding is the rest of the package. Matt is an awesome guy!

Wednesday, December 16, 2015

Dear Diary,

I just found out I am being promoted at the beginning of the year! Nice salary increase and a bigger office! I am thrilled. The office Christmas party is Friday afternoon. All the promotions will be announced then. Matt will be attending the office party with me. I can't wait to tell him.

It is so nice to have someone special to share my big news with. He will more than likely suggest a celebratory dinner tonight at my favorite restaurant. I love this man so much!

Tonight he wanted to talk about our Christmas plans. He has agreed to attend all the Christmas parties I want him to. I want to show him off to my friends. It would be nice to have an engagement ring on my finger when I introduce him but ... I don't think it's that far away, actually. A proposal. I know Matt's proposal will be romantic and over the top.

I'm jumping ahead. We haven't even talked about marriage yet. I haven't been married, and Matt's marriage didn't turn out so well. I don't think it has soured him on marriage. I do think he is probably more cautious about diving into a committed relationship again. He did tell me he hasn't been in a committed relationship since his divorce.

I feel very committed to this relationship and to Matt. I think Matt is committed to our relationship as well. At least, he told me he wasn't dating anyone else at this time. That doesn't mean he is committed to our relationship. It just means he isn't dating anyone else at this time.

I wonder. Is he ready for another relationship? A serious, committed relationship? He hasn't dated since his divorce. Why hasn't he? Why hasn't he dated? I think he said it has been over a year. Will he want to date other women now that he has started to date again?

I think for now I will let it be. I need to stay in the present and enjoy what we have rather than jump ahead to marriage and happily-ever-after.

Monday, January 4, 2016

Dear Diary,

Best Christmas and New Year's EVER!

On Friday the 18th of December, Matt wanted to go for an early dinner. At dinner, he gave me my Christmas present. A European holiday! I had two hours to pack for 16 days! Matt said that whatever I forgot, we could purchase in Europe. (Fortunately, I had a passport.)

What an incredible holiday we had! We traveled by plane, boat, train, car, and even donkeys. We saw museums, temples, castles, and oh so much more! Spain, France, Belgium, Luxembourg, Switzerland, and Italy all in 16 days!

It's amazing how well Matt and I get along. We travel very well together. We have so many of the same likes. He knew exactly what would interest me and planned everything based on my likes! How incredibly romantic!

Now I know what Stephanie and Roger experience when they are with each other. I have never been cherished before and now I am.

If this is a dream, don't wake me. I know, though, that it isn't a dream. I know it is real. I could easily spend the rest of my life with Matt and hope that I do. He is sweet, kind, intelligent, gracious, mannered, has substance and depth, and is charming ... all in one handsome package. How extremely lucky I feel!

Today was also an exciting day at work. Moved into my new office that has a view of downtown and the harbor. It was fun settling into the new position.

Having dinner with Stephanie tomorrow night. Way cool!

Wednesday, January 6, 2016

Dear Diary,

Last night Stephanie and I had dinner. I showed her all the photos I took of our trip. She has decided that the two of us need to go to Paris for a holiday next summer. Told her we could let Matt and Roger tag along.

How fun that would be, the four of us vacationing in Europe together. I have never traveled with another couple before. The four of us are such good friends I think we would have a blast.

Speaking of Matt, I've only had one text this week from him. Monday was his first day back at work as well after our two-week European trip.

Friday, January 8, 2016

Dear Diary,

Haven't seen Matt all week. I texted Matt this morning that I wanted to bring dinner over to his home tonight. He responded with one word, "Great."

I don't think I'll cook. I think I will pick up dinner somewhere. Rather spend the time chatting with him than focusing on a pot on the stove and a dish in the oven.

Saturday, January 9, 2016

Dear Diary,

What did I do wrong? I don't get it. I don't get it. I've cried a bucket full of tears since seeing Matt last night. Notice the paper is a little wet? That's from my tears! And they aren't tears of joy.

Dinner went really well last night. Then he told me Monday he received his next assignments. He said he had a meeting with his boss, the Motivational Speaker. He was given a bonus for the work he did last year and a promotion to Senior Event Manager. He's now in charge of the sales and marketing staff for two different events, one in June and one in November.

I was beaming with happiness for him. A bonus and promotion was great. I had a smile from ear to ear. I was very proud of him.

He told me he leaves tomorrow (which is today) and basically will be gone for the next 11 months. Once the event concludes in one city, he begins everything again in the second city. I told him we could make it work. Between cell phones, messaging, emails, and planes, we could make our relationship eventful and fun.

He told me being promoted and being in charge of the staff, he would have very little time for anything else other than work. It's his responsibility to fill the events with thousands of people and make sure the event comes off without any problems. To perform his duties, he would not have time for a relationship.

I stared at him. "What?" I said. "Even though you will be gone most of this year, we can make this work. I can fly to meet you on the weekends when I'm not working."

He told me I wasn't hearing him. His job was his priority. Showing his boss and his team he was able to handle the new responsibilities, he did not have the time or energy to put into a relationship. I still was confused. Ending our relationship was not anywhere in my thinking.

Finally he said, "I just don't have time for a relationship at this time. You are wonderful. I've had a great time with you. Ending our relationship is not about you. I have to put my energy into my new responsibilities."

It finally sunk into my head and heart. My eyes filled with tears. His compassion and concern for me was confusing. He was concerned about me but still ending our relationship? I didn't understand how come he couldn't do both. I didn't know what to say or do. I think I went into shock.

I don't know how long I sat in silence, motionless, unable to move. Matt asked me if I was okay to drive home or would it be better for him to drive me home?

I shook my head no, stood up, found my purse and keys, and walked out the door. I don't remember driving home. I don't know how long I sat on my couch, motionless, trying to figure out what just happened. I was so exhausted that I curled up on the couch.

A knock on the door woke me up. I was so groggy and dazed, it took me a while to realize that someone was at my door. Was it morning? Still night? The knocking didn't stop. I wondered if it was Matt and he had changed his mind. Did I want it to be Matt? Would I take him back if it was Matt?

I sat up, stood, ran my fingers through my hair, and through the glass pane in the door I could see Stephanie standing at my front door.

Stephanie has been here the last 5 hours. She arrived at 9 a.m. So, it was morning. I slept on my couch last night. Never made it to the bedroom or my bed.

Matt called Roger this morning to say good-bye. Roger asked about the relationship with me. Matt explained to Roger he just didn't have time for a new relationship with the new, added responsibilities of his job. As soon as Roger told Stephanie, Stephanie was on her way over to see me.

My heart is breaking. I thought I met Mr. Right. I guess I was wrong. I don't know what I did wrong. Was I not Ms. Right for Matt? Would he miss me in a couple of weeks and want to rekindle the relationship? If he did, would I want to rekindle the relationship? Obviously, I'm not the priority in his life. Ouch.

Stephanie did her best today to help me understand. The pain is too raw to process or even understand. She tried her best. I think the reality is finally setting in. My Mr. Right was not Mr. Right after all.

Going back to sleep now.

Sunday, January 24, 2016

Dear Diary,

Well, I've slept enough in the last two weeks that today Stephanie asked me if I was hibernating or in a contest with Rip Van Winkle to see who could sleep the most.

Stephanie showed up bright and early yesterday and told me she missed our friendship and we were going to tap. She reminded me that at the class we took the instructor had told us that when two people tap together, the synergy of the energy helps to process what we may not be able to do on our own. I certainly have not been able to process on my own. I've been a hermit since Matt ended our relationship. BTW, no, I have not heard from Matt nor do I think I will.

Stephanie had me tap "Even though:

* The relationship with Matt ended
* I feel like I did something wrong
* I can't pull myself out of my funk
* I don't understand what happened with Matt
* I was not a priority for Matt
* I'm not able to move forward
* I wasn't good enough or important to Matt

* I feel dead inside
* My heart is broken beyond repair
* Death would be easier than this pain
* My heart has been shattered into pieces
* I'm on an emotional roller coaster
* I don't know how to heal the hurt I feel

I totally and completely accept myself.

The instructor had also told us that the day or two after tapping, after integration had taken place, we would begin to feel better. Today, I do feel like I can move on and leave Matt in my past.

Today I called another good friend. She treated me to brunch at a very expensive café. I felt deserving, loved, and cherished. How could I have forgotten that I was deserving and loved?

How thankful I am for the friends that I have. Without them I might still be home feeling sorry for myself, unable to piece my broken heart back together by myself.

# BELIEFS

**Everything in our life is a direct result of our beliefs.**

**A belief** is a mental acceptance of and conviction in the truth, actuality, or validity of something. It is what we believe to be true, whether it is Truth or not. A belief is a thought that influences energy, whether that be our actions or reaction, all the time.

**A mis-belief, a dysfunctional belief** is a belief that takes us away from peace, joy, love, stability, acceptance, and harmony. It causes us to feel stressed, fearful, anxious, and/or insecure.

The reason we aren't successful, happy, or prosperous has to do with our beliefs. Our beliefs determine our thoughts and feelings. Our thoughts and feelings determine our choices and decisions as well as our actions and reactions. Beliefs, then, precede all of our thoughts, feelings, choices, decisions, actions, reactions, and experiences.

> Beliefs **precede** all of our thoughts, feelings, decisions, choices, actions, reactions, and experiences…

> Our beliefs **determine** our thoughts. Our thoughts **determine** our feelings. Our thoughts and feelings **determine** our choices and decisions. Our thoughts and feelings **determine** our actions and reactions.

Can you determine someone's beliefs from their actions and reactions? Persons A, B, C, and D just received a compliment that they looked nice today.

**Person A** responds: "Oh, I don't think so. I so disagree with you."

**Person B** responds: "My hair is a mess. I couldn't do anything with it today."

**Person C** responds: "Okay. What do you want?"

**Person D** responds: "Thank you!"

**Person A**: Totally disagrees. They don't think they look nice today. Person A definitely has self-esteem and self-worth issues. When we are not able to accept a compliment, it's a slap in the face for the person giving the compliment. It's as if Person A is saying, "If you think I look nice, your opinion sucks."

**Person B**: Cannot nor will not accept the compliment. They defect the compliment with a reason why they couldn't look nice. They justify their reason for not accepting the compliment. Think there might be a little bit of anger and/or shame in this type of response?

**Person C**: They think there are strings attached to the compliment. Anyone that would compliment them must want something. Might trust and discernment be an issue for them?

**Person D**: Well, if the response is genuine, then we know they have a healthy self-esteem and self-worth. If the response was said with arrogance, like "Naturally I look nice today" then we could either have someone who really is arrogant or someone who is insecure and using arrogance to hide the insecurity.

Beliefs **precede** all of our actions and reactions, thoughts and feelings, choices and decisions.

# Subconscious Mind

**The Conscious Mind**

The conscious mind is that part of us that thinks, passes judgments, makes decisions, remembers, analyzes, has desires, and communicates with others. It is responsible for logic and reasoning, understanding and comprehension. The mind determines our actions, feelings, thoughts, judgments, and decisions **based on the beliefs.**

**The Subconscious Mind**

The subconscious is the part of the mind that is responsible for all of our involuntary actions like heart beat and breathing rate. It does not evaluate, make decisions, or pass judgment. It just is. It does not determine if something is "right" or "wrong."

> **Our beliefs and memories are stored in the subconscious.**

The subconscious is much like the software of a computer. On the computer keyboard, if we press the key for the letter "a," we will see the letter "a" on the screen, even though we may have wanted to see "t."

Just as a computer can only do what it has been programmed to do, we can only do as we are programmed to do. Our programming is determined by our beliefs.

> **If we want to make changes in our lives, we have to change the programming, the mis-beliefs in the subconscious.**

# 3 Rules of the Subconscious Mind

Three rules of the subconscious mind include:

1. **Personal**. It only understands "I," "me," "myself." First person.

2. **Positive**. The subconscious does not hear the word "no." When you say, "I am not going to eat that piece of cake," the subconscious mind hears "Yummm! Cake! I am going to eat a piece of that cake!"

3. **Present time**. Time does not exist for the subconscious. The only time it knows is "now," present time. "I'm going to start my diet tomorrow." "Tomorrow" never comes thus the diet is never started.

# Emotional Freedom Technique

If we want to make changes in our lives, long-lasting, permanent, constructive changes, we have to change the destructive, dysfunctional, misbeliefs in the subconscious. We have to change the programming in the subconscious.

**EFT Tapping allows us to change the dysfunctional, destructive, misbeliefs on a subconscious level.**

## What is EFT – Emotional Freedom Technique

EFT is a technique that allows us to change dysfunctional beliefs and emotions on a subconscious level. It involves making a statement while tapping different points along meridian paths.

The general principle behind EFT is that the cause of all negative emotions is a disruption in the body's energy system. By tapping on locations where a number of the different meridians flow, we are able to release unproductive memories, emotions, and beliefs which cause the blockages.

## EFT Tapping Statements:

An EFT statement has three parts to it:

Part 1: Starts with "Even though," followed by

Part 2: A statement which could be the dysfunctional emotion or belief, and

Part 3: Ends with "I totally and completely accept myself."

So, a total statement would be "Even though, I fear change, I totally and completely accept myself."

(1) "Even though..." statement 3 times — Karate chop
(2) Statement
(3) "Completely totally accept myself"
(4) Tap the 'statement' on all points

Take a deep breath

# How to Tap Short Form of EFT – Emotional Freedom Technique

The instructions below are described if you were using your right hand. Reverse directions to tap using the left hand. It is only necessary to tap one side. Tapping both sides does not add any additional benefit.

## I. Begin with circling:

A. With the fingertips of your right hand, find a tender spot below your left collar bone. Once you have found the tender spot, with your right fingertips, press firmly on the spot, make a circular motion toward the left shoulder, toward the outside, clockwise.

B. As your fingers are circling and pressing against the tender spot, make the following statement 3 times: "Even though,___[mis-belief statement]___, I totally and completely accept myself." An example would be: "Even though, I fear change, I totally and completely accept myself."

## II. Tapping:

A. After the third time, tap the following 8 points repeating the [mis-belief statement] each time with each point. Tap each point 7 – 10 times:

1. The inner edge of the eyebrow just above the eye. [I fear change.]

2. Temple, just to the side of the eye. [I fear change.]

3. Just below the eye (on the cheekbone). [I fear change.]

4. Under the nose. [I fear change.]

5. Under the lips. [I fear change.]

6. Under the knob of the inside edge of the collar bone. [I fear change.]

7. 3" under the arm pit. [I fear change.]

8. Top back of the head. [I fear change.]

B. After tapping, take a deep breath. If you are not able to take a deep, full, satisfying breath, do eye rolls.

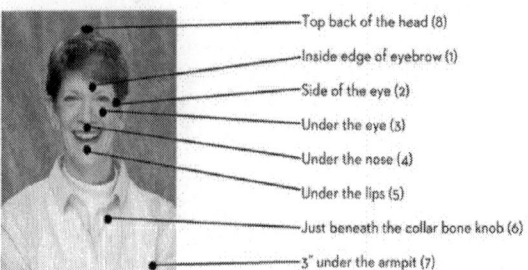

## III. Eye rolls

A. With one hand, tap continuously on the **back** of the other hand between the 4th and 5th fingers.

B. Head is held straight forward, eyes looking straight down.

C. For 6 seconds, roll your eyes from the floor straight up toward the ceiling while repeating the statement. Keep the head straight forward, only moving the eyes.

## IV. Take another deep breath.

## Yawning and Taking a Deep Breath

From Oriental medicine, we know that when Chi (energy) flows freely through the meridians, the body is healthy and balanced. Physical, mental, and/or emotional illness can result when the energy is blocked.

Dysfunctional beliefs and emotions produce blocks along the meridians, blocking energy from flowing freely in the body.

With EFT tapping, as we tap we are releasing the blocks. As blocked energy is able to flow more freely, the body is now able to "breathe a sigh of relief." Yawning is that sigh of relief.

If, after tapping, we are able to take a complete, deep, full, and satisfying breath, we know that an EFT tapping statement has cleared. This yawn is an indication that an EFT tapping statement has cleared.

If the yawn or breath is not a full, deep breath then the statement didn't clear completely.

## Integration...What Happens After Tapping

After tapping, our system needs some downtime for integration to take place. When the physical body and the mind are "idle," integration can then take place.

Sometimes, in the first 24 hours after tapping, we might find ourselves vegging more than normal, sleeping more than normal, or more tired than normal. This downtime is needed to integrate the new changes.

After installing a new program into our computer, sometimes we have to reboot the computer (shut down and restart) for the new program to be integrated into the system.

After tapping, our bodies need to reboot. We need some downtime. When we sleep, the new changes are integrated.

Healing begins naturally after the body has had a chance to integrate.

Sometimes after tapping, we forget the intensity of our pain and think that our feeling better had nothing to do with the tapping. Something so simple could not possibly create the improvement in our state of mind!

When we cut our finger, once it is healed, we don't even remember cutting our finger. As we move toward health, wealth, and well-being, sometimes we don't remember how unhappy, restless, or isolated we once felt.

# How Does EFT Tapping Work?

1. **Acceptance:** The last part of the tapping statement we say, "I totally and completely accept myself." **Acceptance brings us into present time.** We can only heal if we are in present time. Laughter brings us into present time. "Laughter is the best medicine."

2. **Addresses the current mis-belief on a subconscious level:** In order to make changes in our lives, we have to change the dysfunctional beliefs, the mis-belief on a subconscious level. The middle part of the tapping statements are the "instructions" for the subconscious. **In order to made changes in our lives, we only care what the subconscious hears.**

3. **Pattern interrupt:** Dysfunctional memories and/or mis-beliefs disrupt or block the flow of energy from flowing freely along the meridians. Tapping is a pattern interrupt that disrupts the flow of energy to allow our **body's own Infinite Wisdom to come forth for healing.**

4. **Mis-direct:** One role of the physical body is to protect us. When our hand is too close to a flame, the body automatically pulls the hand back to safety. An EFT Tapping statement that agrees with the current belief is more effective. The physical body is less likely to "sabotage" the tapping if it agrees with the current belief.

**An Example:** The very first tapping statement we need to tap is: "It is not okay or safe for my life to change." Even though our lives are constantly changing does not mean we are comfortable or okay with change. When we are not comfortable with change, it creates stress for the body.

EFT Tapping Statement: "It is not okay or safe for my life to change."

* This statement appeases the physical body since it agrees with the current belief.

* The subconscious hears, "It is okay and safe for my life to change."

* The tapping disrupts the energy flow so our Truth can come forth.

The body will always gravitate to health, wealth, and well-being when the conditions allow it. Tapping weeds the garden so that the blossoms can bloom more easily and effortlessly.

# SCIENCE AND EFT TAPPING RESEARCH

EFT has been researched in more than 10 countries by more than 60 investigators whose results have been published in more than 20 different peer-reviewed journals. Two of the leading researchers are Dawson Church, Ph.D. and David Feinstein, Ph.D.

Dr. Dawson Church, a leading expert on energy psychology and an EFT master, has gathered all the research information and can be found on this website: www.EFTUniverse.com.

## Two Research Studies Discussed Below

### Harvard Medical Schools Studies and the Brain's Stress Response

Studies at the Harvard Medical School revealed that stimulating the body's meridian points significantly reduced activity in a part of the brain called the amygdala.

The amygdala can be thought of as the body's alarm system. When the body is experiencing trauma or fear, the amygdala is triggered and the body is flooded with cortisol also known as the "stress hormone." The stress response sets up an intricate chain reaction.

The studies showed that stimulating or tapping points along the meridians such as EFT tapping, drastically reduced and/or eliminated the stress response and the resulting chain reaction.

### Dr. Dawson Church and Cortisol Reduction

Another significant study was conducted by Dr. Dawson Church. He studied the impact an hour tapping session would have on the cortisol levels of 83 subjects. He also measured the cortisol levels of people who received traditional talk therapy and the cortisol levels of a third group who received no treatment at all.

On an average, for the 83 subjects that completed an hour tapping session, cortisol levels were reduced by 24% reduction. Some subjects experienced a 50% reduction in cortisol levels.

Subjects that completed an hour long traditional talk therapy and the subjects that had completed neither sessions did not experience any significant cortisol reduction.

# Benefits of Using EFT Tapping

\* The last part of the statement is "I totally and completely **accept** myself." **Acceptance** brings us into present time. Healing can only take place when we are in present time.

\* By tapping, we are **calling forth our truths**. The key word here is "**our**." Not anyone else's. If my name is "Lucas," tapping the statement "Even though my name is Troy," my name will not be changed to Troy.

\* Tapping **calls forth our own body's Infinite Wisdom**. When we cut our finger, our body knows how to heal the cut itself. Once the dysfunctional emotions, experiences, and beliefs have been "deleted," our body **automatically** gravitates to health, wealth, wisdom, peace, love, joy…

\* By changing the mis-beliefs and dysfunctional emotions on a subconscious level, the changes we make with EFT are **permanent.**

\* By tapping, we are "**neutralizing**" the stored memories that have been blocking energy from flowing freely along the meridians.

\* Another benefit of tapping and EFT is desensitization. Let's say, we have a difficult person in our life that ignores us and/or criticizes us and we tap the statement: "This difficult person [or their name] ignores and criticizes me."

**Tapping doesn't mean they will no longer ignore and/or criticize us.**

It can, though, **desensitize us** so we no longer are affected by their behavior. Once we are desensitized, our perception and mental thinking improves, we are better able to make informed decisions, we don't take and make everything personally, our health is not negatively impacted, our heart doesn't beat 100 beats/minute, smoke stops coming out of our ears, and our faces don't turn red with anger and frustration.

# The Very First EFT Tapping Statement to Tap

The very first EFT tapping statement I have clients and students tap is "It is not okay or safe for my life to change." I have muscle tested this statement with more than a thousand people. Not one person tested strong that is was okay or safe for their life to change.

**How effective can EFT or any therapy be if it isn't okay or safe for our lives to change?**

Since our lives are constantly changing, if it is not okay or safe for our lives to change, every time our lives change, it creates stress for the body. Stress creates another whole set of issues for ourselves and our lives.

## Intensity Level

One measure of knowing how much an "issue" has been "resolved" is to begin, before tapping, by giving the issue an intensity number between 1 – 10, with 10 being high.

For example, you want a romantic partnership yet, you haven't met "the one." Thinking about the likelihood of a romantic relationship happening for you, how likely, on a scale of 1 – 10, with 10 being very likely and 1, not likely at all, would a romantic relationship happen for you?

Okay. You gave yourself a 2. Now let's start tapping!

When asked what the "issues" might be, "Well," you say. "It doesn't seem as if the people I want, want me."

Great tapping statement. So, you tap out, "Even though, the people I want don't want me, I totally and completely accept myself." After tapping you check in with yourself, the Intensity Level (IL) has gone up to a 4, a little bit more likely.

What comes to mind now? You say, "No one will find me desirable." Great tapping statement. You tap out, "Even though, no one will find me desirable, I totally and completely accept myself." Check the IL. How likely? Now you are at a 5. Cool! Progress.

What comes to mind now? You say, "I'm not comfortable being vulnerable in romantic relationships." Great tapping statement. You tap out, "Even though, I'm not comfortable being vulnerable in a romantic relationship, I totally and completely accept myself." Check the IL. Now it is a 6. Still progress.

What comes to mind now? "Well, it feels like if I am in a relationship, I will lose a lot of my freedom." Make this into a tapping statements. "Even though, I will lose my freedom when I am in a relationship, I totally and completely accept myself." The IL has gone up to a 7.

What comes to mind now? "Oh, if I was in a relationship, I would have to be accountable to someone!" Make this into a tapping statement: "Even though,

I would have to be accountable to someone if I was in a relationship, I totally and completely accept myself." Wow...the IL is 9, very likely!

GIVING AN ISSUE AN INTENSITY LEVEL GIVES US AN INDICATION OF THE PROGRESS WE ARE MAKING WITH RESOLVING AND/OR HEALING THAT ISSUE IN OUR LIVES.

# Using a Negative EFT Tapping Statement

Our beliefs **precede** all of our thoughts, feelings, decisions, choices, actions, reactions, and experiences…

If we want to make changes in our lives, we have to change the mis-beliefs, the dysfunctional beliefs. Our beliefs are stored in the subconscious.

To change our lives, to change a belief, we only care what the subconscious hears when we tap. The subconscious does not hear the word "no." When we say, "I am not going to eat that piece of cake," the subconscious hears, "Yummm, cake!"

Example, if we don't believe we had what it takes to be successful and we tap the statement, "I have what it takes to be successful," the body could sabotage the tapping. We could tap and it won't clear.

If instead the statement we make is "I don't have what it takes to be successful," the "**not**" appeases the physical body and the subconscious hears, "I have what it takes to be successful!"

# Finishing Touches (Optional)

One way to finish this eBook is to tap positive statements. The following 16 statements can be completed in two rounds of tapping, stating one statement for each tapping location.

**Eyebrow** – All is well in my life.

**Temple** – Every day in every way I am getting better and better.

**Under the Eye** – I am fulfilled in every way, every day.

**Under the Nose** – My blessings appears in rich appropriate form with divine timing.

**Under the Lips** – I am an excellent steward of wealth and am blessed with great abundance.

**Collarbone Knob** – I take complete responsibility for everything in my life.

**Under the Arm** – I have all the tools, skills, and abilities to excel in my life.

**Top back part of the Head** – I know I will be able to handle anything that arises in my life.

**Eyebrow** – All my dreams, hopes, wishes, and goals are being fulfilled each and every day.

**Temple** – Divine love expressing through me, now draws to me new ideas.

**Under the Eye** – I am comfortable with my life changing.

**Under the Nose** – I bless the increase in my health, wealth, and happiness.

**Under the Lips** – I know what needs to be done and follow through to completion.

**Collarbone Knob** – My health is perfect in every way, physically, mentally, emotionally, and spiritually.

*Jesus*

**Under the Arm** – I invite into my subconscious Archangel Raphael to heal all that needs to be forgiven, released, and redeemed. Cleanse me and free me from it now.   *St. Archangel Raphael pray for me*

**Top back part of the Head** – The light of God surrounds me. The love of God enfolds me. The power of God protects me. The presence of God watches over and flows through me.

# How to Use This Book

1. The statements are divided into sections. Read through the statements in one section. As you read a statement, notice if you have any reaction to the statement or feel the statement might be true for you. If so, note the number for that statement.

2. Once you have completed reading all the statements in one section, go back and reread the statements you noted and rate them on a scale of 1 – 10, with 10 being a biggie."

3. List the top statements.

4. From this list, select one and describe how it plays out in your life. It is important to recognize and identify the pattern. What are the consequences of having this mis-belief? Is there a trigger? How does it begin? How does it benefit you? How has it harmed you? There will be a different example listed in each section.

5. Tap out the statements. Statements can be combined for scripts...a different statement on each of the different tapping points in one round of tapping.

6. Describe any flashbacks or memories that you might have had as you were tapping out the statements. Describe any ah-has, insights, and/or thoughts you might have had as a result of tapping the statements.

7. After tapping all the statements, review them to determine if you still have a reaction to any of the statements. If you do, you have several options. One, put a "Why" before the statement. Tap out the answer. Secondly, note that this statement may not have cleared and continue on to the next section. Most likely, after additional statements are tapped, statements that may not have cleared, will clear without having to tap the statement again.

8. Allow some downtime for integration and for the body to heal.

9. The number of sections you do at a time will be up to you. Initially, you might want to do one section to determine if you get tired and need to have some downtime after tapping.

10. The day after tapping, again review the statements you tapped to

determine if you still have a reaction. If you do, follow the instructions in #7.

# Tapping Statements 1 – 20

*Hiding in my room, safe within my womb, I touch no one and no one touches me. I am a rock, I am an island. And a rock feels no pain; And an island never cries.*

*Paul Simon*
*From song I Am a Rock*

1. I use (fill in the 3 most destructive from the following) *alcohol, sugar, caffeine, over/under eating, excessive spending, drugs, nicotine, binge eating, promiscuity, chocolate, too much sleep, too little sleep, TV watching, and/or computer games* to numb the pain I feel.

2. I miss "us."

3. I'm not lovable.

4. I am undesirable.

5. I feel dead inside.

6. I can't stop crying.

7. I feel empty inside.

8. I'm not able to sleep.

9. I've lost a part of me.

10. I'm not able to focus.

11. I'm not good enough.

12. The future looks grim.

13. I will always be alone.

14. I'm mentally depleted.

15. Life isn't worth living.

16. I don't laugh anymore.

17. They are irreplaceable.

18. The tears seem endless.

19. None of it makes sense.
20. My pain will never end.

# Journaling Page for Statements 1 – 20

*When we hold someone responsible for what we experience, we lose power. When we depend upon another person for the experiences we think are necessary to our well-being, we live continually in the fear that they will not deliver.*

*Gary Zukav*

1. From the tapping statements in this section 1 – 20, list the top seven statements that you thought or felt applied to you:

2. From this list of seven statements, select one and describe how it plays out in your life. Give an example or two. It is important to recognize and identify the pattern. Is there a trigger? How does it begin? How has it benefited you? How has it harmed you? For instance, do you just want to stay home alone and hide under the covers? Do you have the tools and skills that a friendship/relationship would require? Or is it that you select the wrong people to befriend and end up used and abused? Hiding is about avoidance. What are you avoiding?

3. Tap out the top 7 statements.

4. As you were tapping out the statements, did you have any flashback or memories of the past, any additional insights, and/or ah-ha thoughts? If so, write them down. Make note of them.

# Tapping Statements 21 – 40

*Relationships are like glass. Sometimes it's better to leave them broken than try to hurt yourself putting them back together.*

*Anonymous*

21. My grief will go on forever.
22. I miss who I was with them.
23. I don't want to feel the pain.
24. I'm more cynical than usual.
25. Life is too painful to endure.
26. I will never be good enough.
27. I cannot go on without them.
28. It still makes no sense to me.
29. I feel unloved and unwanted.
30. I often feel inferior to others.
31. My life is over without them.
32. Nothing seems real anymore.
33. It's not safe to be vulnerable.
34. I'm not relationship material.
35. I isolated myself from others.
36. My mood changes constantly.
37. I'm not taking care of myself.
38. My self-worth is non-existent.
39. I have emotionally shut down.
40. I feel worthless and unlovable.

# Journaling Page for Statements 21 – 40

*If you are going through hell, keep going.*

Rob Estes

1. From the tapping statements in this section 1 – 20, list the top seven statements that you thought or felt applied to you:

2. From this list of seven statements, select one and describe how it plays out in your life. Give an example or two. It is important to recognize and identify the pattern. Is there a trigger? How does it begin? How has it benefited you? How has it harmed you? For instance, you can't let go of the pain. When we can't or won't let go of the pain, we benefit in some way. Holding onto the pain, might be about avoiding another relationship. Might be we want to blame them for our abandonment rather than look at our role in the relationship. Might be we would rather stay angry than move on with our life. How does holding onto the pain serve you?

3. Tap out the top 7 statements.

4. As you were tapping out the statements, did you have any flashback or memories of the past, any additional insights, and/or ah-ha thoughts? If so, write them down. Make note of them.

# Tapping Statements 41 – 60

*Grief is like the ocean. It comes on waves ebbing and flowing. Sometimes the water is calm and sometimes it is overwhelming. All we can do is learn to swim.*

*Vicki Harrison*

41. I will always be broken.
42. Life is hostile and cruel.
43. Life seems meaningless.
44. I'm undeserving of love.
45. I'm tired of the struggle.
46. I wish I could disappear.
47. I feel physically drained.
48. I'm barely surviving life.
49. The future is dead for me.
50. No one will ever love me.
51. I'm drowning in self-pity.
52. I don't enjoy life anymore.
53. I lost me when I lost them.
54. I've lost interest in my life.
55. I will never be happy again.
56. It's unbearable being alone.
57. I can't stop asking, "Why?"
58. I will never find love again.
59. I'm unhappy and miserable.
60. I miss the life I used to live.

# Journaling Page for Statements 41 – 60

*Nothing is terminal, just transitional.*

*Dr. Robert Schuller*

1. From the tapping statements in this section 1 – 20, list the top seven statements that you thought or felt applied to you:

2. From this list of seven statements, select one and describe how it plays out in your life. Give an example or two. It is important to recognize and identify the pattern. Is there a trigger? How does it begin? How has it benefited you? How has it harmed you? For instance, are you incomplete now that they are gone? Are they gone because you are incomplete? What would happen if you were complete all by yourself? Do you think you would not need anyone or that anyone would need you?

3. Tap out the top 7 statements.

4. As you were tapping out the statements, did you have any flashback or memories of the past, any additional insights, and/or ah-ha thoughts? If so, write them down. Make note of them.

# Tapping Statements 61 – 80

*A lot of people say they want to get out of pain, but they aren't willing to make healing a high priority. They aren't willing to look inside to see the source of their pain in order to deal with it.*

*Lindsay Wagner*

61. I'm stuck in a very dark place.
62. I've lost interest in everything.
63. My life feels hopeless and flat.
64. I avoid socializing with others.
65. I sleep to avoid consciousness.
66. I have no inner sense of worth.
67. My life is empty without them.
68. I'm helpless to change my life.
69. I don't know how to start over.
70. I lack the ability to attract love.
71. I can't shake the sadness I feel.
72. I stay in bed to escape the pain.
73. My self-esteem is non-existent.
74. I don't know what I did wrong.
75. I still question if I am to blame.
76. I miss their presence in my life.
77. I'm having difficulty accepting.
78. I'm having difficulty letting go.
79. My downward spiral is endless.
80. I analyze so I don't have to feel.

# Journaling Page for Statements 61 – 80

*People are lonely because they build walls instead of bridges.*

J. F. Newton

1. From the tapping statements in this section 1 – 20, list the top seven statements that you thought or felt applied to you:

2. From this list of seven statements, select one and describe how it plays out in your life. Give an example or two. It is important to recognize and identify the pattern. Is there a trigger? How does it begin? How has it benefited you? How has it harmed you? For instance, no matter how much you want to be with someone, no one wants you. Our reality has a tendency to follow our thoughts. What we focus on, expands. When we focus on what we don't want, we get more of what we don't want. When we focus on what we want, we have a tendency to gravitate towards that which we want. A healthy person is not attracted to someone that doesn't have confidence in themselves. What issue needs to be healed to create the reality and the relationship you desire?

3. Tap out the top 7 statements.

4. As you were tapping out the statements, did you have any flashback or memories of the past, any additional insights, and/or ah-ha thoughts? If so, write them down. Make note of them.

# Tapping Statements 81 – 100

*The first and greatest form of courage is the courage to take responsible for our own life. Like it or not, we alone are responsible for the person we are today, the state of our heart, and the shape of our life. We can point our finger 'til the cows come home, but at the end of the day, the buck stops with us.*

*Margie Warrell*

81. I feel a heavy weight on my chest.
82. I have waves of sadness and tears.
83. Life doesn't make sense anymore.
84. My body and mind ache for them.
85. I feel discouraged and abandoned.
86. Painful reminders are everywhere.
87. I can't pull myself out of my grief.
88. I'm not able to get on with my life.
89. My mind feels heavy and clouded.
90. I'm on an emotional roller-coaster.
91. I constantly feel tired and fatigued.
92. I'm not special enough to be loved.
93. I know I will never be happy again.
94. I start crying when I least expect it.
95. My self-esteem has been destroyed.
96. I negate and neglect my own needs.
97. I don't want to go on without them.
98. It's pointless to take care of myself.
99. Nothing ever turns out right for me.
100. Being alone feels like a punishment.

# Journaling Page for Statements 81 – 100

*Experience is a hard teacher. She gives the test first, the lesson afterwards.*

*Vernon Sanders Law*

1. From the tapping statements in this section 1 – 20, list the top seven statements that you thought or felt applied to you:

2. From this list of seven statements, select one and describe how it plays out in your life. Give an example or two. It is important to recognize and identify the pattern. Is there a trigger? How does it begin? How has it benefited you? How has it harmed you? For instance, do you keep intimate relationships at arm's length? Is this to stay "safe?" Ships are safe in the harbor but that is not what ships are for. We are not meant to be an island all unto ourselves. Do you know how to do intimate relationships successfully? Do you have the tools and skills to have a successful intimate relationship?

3. Tap out the top 7 statements.

4. As you were tapping out the statements, did you have any flashback or memories of the past, any additional insights, and/or ah-ha thoughts? If so, write them down. Make note of them.

# Tapping Statements 101 – 120

*Your biggest problem or difficulty today has been sent to you at this moment to teach you something you need to know to be happier and more successful in the future.*

*Brian Tracy*

101. I feel as if I am coming unglued.
102. I have a constant sense of doom.
103. I'm short-tempered and irritable.
104. I've withdrawn from everything.
105. The relationship is irreplaceable.
106. I feel lonely, alone, and unloved.
107. I'm to blame for my painful loss.
108. I miss the life I was going to live.
109. I wake up tired, anxious, and sad.
110. My confidence is down the drain.
111. I don't know how to find closure.
112. I'm not good enough to be loved.
113. I'm more indecisive than normal.
114. I feel lost, unable to find my way.
115. I can't stop talking about my loss.
116. I have no control over my moods.
117. My heart is broken beyond repair.
118. I have nothing to look forward to.
119. I can't move past this devastation.
120. My broken heart will never mend.

# Journaling Page for Statements 101 – 120

*Sometimes I wish I were a kid again. Skinned knees are a lot easier to fix than a broken heart.*

*Unknown*

1. From the tapping statements in this section 1 – 20, list the top seven statements that you thought or felt applied to you:

2. From this list of seven statements, select one and describe how it plays out in your life. Give an example or two. It is important to recognize and identify the pattern. Is there a trigger? How does it begin? How has it benefited you? How has it harmed you? For instance, do you lack the energy to move forward in your life? Do you know what you want to do? Have you created anything compelling to move toward? Are you afraid you might fail? Is it easier to stay in apathy rather than to learn new skills, to find meaning for your life, and/or to energize your life?

3. Tap out the top 7 statements.

4. As you were tapping out the statements, did you have any flashback or memories of the past, any additional insights, and/or ah-ha thoughts? If so, write them down. Make note of them.

# Tapping Statements 121 – 140

*"Buttons" are old emotional wounds crying out for healing. When everything seems to be going against you, remember that an airplane takes off against the wind, not with it.*

*Henry Ford*

121. My anger has a momentum of its own.
122. I don't know how to let go of my grief.
123. I can't find the joy of living any longer.
124. It's hard to think clearly or concentrate.
125. I'm full of self-doubt and self-loathing.
126. I'm incomplete now that they are gone.
127. I'm totally hopeless and full of despair.
128. I'm sinking in the quicksand of despair.
129. I'm not able to ask for help from others.
130. It is difficult to make it through the day.
131. I don't know how to heal the hurt I feel.
132. I tell others how badly I have been hurt.
133. I feel dazed, confused, and preoccupied.
134. I feel depressed and sad most of the day.
135. I feel irritable and consumed with anger.
136. I don't have the energy to get out of bed.
137. I keep busy so I don't have to remember.
138. I'm not strong enough to risk love again.
139. I'm devastated when a relationship ends.
140. I don't know how to make my life better.

# Journaling Page for Statements 121 – 140

*The more anger towards the past you carry in your heart, the less capable you are of loving in the present.*

*Barbara De Angelis*

1. From the tapping statements in this section 1 – 20, list the top seven statements that you thought or felt applied to you:

2. From this list of seven statements, select one and describe how it plays out in your life. Give an example or two. It is important to recognize and identify the pattern. Is there a trigger? How does it begin? How has it benefited you? How has it harmed you? For instance, is the depression a result of feeling unloved, unlovable, and there will never be anyone that can or will love you? Do you expect someone else to love you when you don't love yourself?

3. Tap out the top 7 statements.

4. As you were tapping out the statements, did you have any flashback or memories of the past, any additional insights, and/or ah-ha thoughts? If so, write them down. Make note of them.

# Tapping Statements 141 – 160

*Having experienced, struggled with, and come to terms with my own particular share of 'necessary losses' over the years, I've come to realize that those losses have taught me some of life's most valuable lessons.*

*Marty Tousley*

141. I am out of strength and confidence.
142. I dread getting out of bed every day.
143. I'm unable to deal with my feelings.
144. Nothing will ever be the same again.
145. I'm addicted to romantic infatuation.
146. My self-confidence has been eroded.
147. I'm tired of hearing "Time heals all."
148. I cannot get over my disappointment.
149. I'm having difficulty letting them go.
150. I deny my pain, guilt, and/or sadness.
151. I've lost my appeal as a sexual being.
152. I don't know how to get to happiness.
153. I don't know how to survive this loss.
154. My life has been turned upside down.
155. I can't get beyond my disappointment.
156. I won't be able to stop crying if I start.
157. I constantly yearn for what I have lost.
158. I'm sinking in the quicksand of inertia.
159. I'm not able to move through the pain.
160. I can't find me now that they are gone.

# Journaling Page for Statements 141 – 160

*There comes a time when the risk to remain tight in a bud will be more painful than the risk it takes to blossom.*

*Anais Nin*

1. From the tapping statements in this section 1 – 20, list the top seven statements that you thought or felt applied to you:

2. From this list of seven statements, select one and describe how it plays out in your life. Give an example or two. It is important to recognize and identify the pattern. Is there a trigger? How does it begin? How has it benefited you? How has it harmed you? For instance, do you deny your pain? What would happen if you acknowledged the pain you have? Would you drown in your pain never to be heard from again? Would you have to deal with your lost hopes and dreams? Would you have to take responsibility for your life?

3. Tap out the top 7 statements.

4. As you were tapping out the statements, did you have any flashback or memories of the past, any additional insights, and/or ah-ha thoughts? If so, write them down. Make note of them.

# Tapping Statements 161 – 180

*A friendship is like sand in your hand: if held loosely in the palm of your hand, it stays there, but as soon as you close your hand tightly, it slips through your fingers.*

*Unknown*

161. I'm afraid to let myself go and feel good.
162. I don't know how to go on without them.
163. I still miss their companionship so much.
164. It's difficult getting through the holidays.
165. My joy died when the relationship ended.
166. I will never be able to heal the hurt I feel.
167. I will end up alone for the rest of my life.
168. I'm shattered that this relationship ended.
169. I feel angry, sad, hurt, broken, and lonely.
170. I still seem to do everything at half speed.
171. I've retreated and withdrawn from others.
172. I stay busy so I don't have to think or feel.
173. I'm angry that the life I knew is no longer.
174. I don't care that I'm not taking care of me.
175. I'm disappointed every time I am hopeful.
176. My brain has been filled up with molasses.
177. My hopes and dreams have been shattered.
178. Life is synonymous with pain and struggle.
179. I feel as if I have been stabbed in the heart.
180. My pain is more than what I can deal with.

# Journaling Page for Statements 161 – 180

*Even a happy life cannot be without a measure of darkness and the word happiness would lose its meaning if it were not balanced by sadness.*

*Carl Jung*

1. From the tapping statements in this section 1 – 20, list the top seven statements that you thought or felt applied to you:

2. From this list of seven statements, select one and describe how it plays out in your life. Give an example or two. It is important to recognize and identify the pattern. Is there a trigger? How does it begin? How has it benefited you? How has it harmed you? For instance, do you feel like a complete failure that this relationship has ended? Stepping back and looking at this person, did they select someone that was capable of loving, not "relationship material" thinking they could fix them, that had a history of healthy relationships? Is the failure they feel a result of whom they selected for a relationship or the actual interaction in the relationship?

3. Tap out the top 7 statements.

4. As you were tapping out the statements, did you have any flashback or memories of the past, any additional insights, and/or ah-ha thoughts? If so, write them down. Make note of them.

# TAPPING STATEMENTS 181 – 200

*The risk of love is loss and the price of loss is grief. But the pain of grief is only a shadow when compared with the pain of never risking love.*

*Hilary Stanton Zunin*

181. I keep busy so I don't have to feel the pain.
182. I wake up with no interest of doing my life.
183. Rejection is evidence of my unlovableness.
184. There is something terribly wrong with me.
185. Life seems meaningless and overwhelming.
186. I focus on my failures and what I did wrong.
187. I keep intimate relationships at arm's length.
188. I don't know what it will take for me to heal.
189. I sacrifice my needs to fulfill someone else's.
190. The failure of the relationship is all my fault.
191. I cannot face or accept being a single person.
192. I attach to my partners with emotional epoxy.
193. I feel detached and disconnected from others.
194. I will drown in my own tears if I feel my pain.
195. I keep old wounds bleeding and from healing.
196. I don't know who I am without a relationship.
197. I feel powerless to change what has happened.
198. I don't know how to get my life back on track.
199. I don't know how to make my life meaningful.
200. My hopes for the future were invested in them.

## Journaling Page for Statements 181 – 200

*Holding onto anger is like grasping a hot coal with the intent of throwing it at someone else. You are the one who gets burned.*

*Buddha*

1. From the tapping statements in this section 1 – 20, list the top seven statements that you thought or felt applied to you:

2. From this list of seven statements, select one and describe how it plays out in your life. Give an example or two. It is important to recognize and identify the pattern. Is there a trigger? How does it begin? How has it benefited you? How has it harmed you? For instance, was your need for love invested in them? Do you love yourself? When we depend on another person for love, we continually live in fear for the day that we will be abandoned because we are not lovable.

3. Tap out the top 7 statements.

4. As you were tapping out the statements, did you have any flashback or memories of the past, any additional insights, and/or ah-ha thoughts? If so, write them down. Make note of them.

Printed in Great Britain
by Amazon